OBAMACARE-PROOF YOUR PRACTICE

The Simple Step-by-Step Plan
to Make More Money,
See Less Patients,
and Practice Medicine
on Your Terms

by Scott R. Cartwright, MPH

1ˢᵗ Edition 2013

Copyright © 2013 by Health Priority, LLC

All rights reserved.

Published by Health Priority, LLC.
7770 Regents Rd. #249, San Diego, CA 92122

Scott Cartwright
7770 Regents Rd. #249, San Diego, CA 92122

Printed in the United States of America

To my wife Mignonne, who always holds my feet to the fire and motivates me in ways she will never know.

To my son Evans, who has made me realize what life is really about. (What's 1 + 1?...)

All courses of action are risky,
so prudence is not in
avoiding danger
- it's impossible -
but calculating risk
and acting decisively.

Make mistakes of ambition
and not mistakes of sloth.
Develop the strength to
do bold things...
not the strength to suffer.

-Niccolo Machiavelli
The Prince

CONTENTS

Introduction

Here's the problem...if you're anything like the doctors I talk to, especially doctors in private practice, you have two major concerns: 1) your ever-increasing overhead and 2) your ever-decreasing reimbursements. In addition, as if these two things weren't enough, you don't like the fact that nowadays insurance companies are running the show. They decide all of the "if's, how's and when's" of your reimbursements and basically you've become an employee of the insurance company.

In addition, you aren't allowed to and you can't practice the kind of medicine you really want to practice. Medicine where you get to spend quality time with your patients, spending more than 10 minutes with them during an office visit, and really getting to know them and their problems, their symptoms, and any other social issues that they may have going on.

Another problem is that you see what's on the horizon. There are more and more private practices being bought up by hospitals and doctors are becoming employees of the hospital. And you definitely don't want this to happen because you realize the freedom you have to give up when you become an employee of the hospital. The bottom line is that you're not getting the income you deserve and you're not getting to practice medicine on your terms.

Unfortunately, things are only going to get worse with Obamacare. As you know, there is already a projected shortage of 40,000 primary care physicians that will be needed to take care of the 32 million new patients covered by Obamacare. These 32 million new patients are going to need to see doctors and the doctors that are currently available are going to be required to see them.

The red tape and administrative burden of Obamacare is a nightmare that is surely keeping you up at night. You're worried about the additional requirements, the regulations, the additional staff that you'll have to hire in order to be compliant...and the list goes on and on. Fortunately, there's a way for you to not have to deal with all of these things or at least minimize the impact that Obamacare has on your private practice.

This book is meant to reveal to you exactly what you need to do so you can 1) attract and treat the types of patients that you really want to care for, 2) take better care of your patients, 3) maximize the efficiency within your practice, 4) generate more revenue from your practice, which allows you to 5) see less patients and take more time off!

All of these things can be done but in order for them to work, you must be willing to implement the concepts from this book.

So let's get to it!

Chapter 1

HOW TO USE
THIS BOOK

I'm going to state the obvious here...so bear with me for a minute. You're a doctor and you're very busy. Time is your most valuable asset and I don't have any intention of wasting your time. Most importantly, this book is certainly not intended to waste your time...quite the contrary. This book is meant to save you time and make you more money!

Now, as the doctor you're the conductor of your symphony. You don't have the time to learn how to play all of the instruments in the orchestra. You're there to conduct. So what I suggest is that you read the rest of this chapter and then Chapters 2, 6, 7, and 9 (in this order), at a minimum, so you can get a good idea of the basics of what is going to happen (or what needs to happen) and then hand this book

1

off to your receptionist, assistant, nurse, or practice manager so he or she can read the whole thing.

I will be addressing you, the doctor, in this book but it's really meant for you to give to a staff member so they can do the action steps. All of the concepts and things that need to be done are found in the book and the actions steps are covered in the Tutorials section found in Chapter 12.

If you or your staff gets stuck anywhere along the way, feel free to give me a call at 858.255.1612 and I'll help you out.

You get to create YOUR masterpiece

The beauty of being the conductor is that the orchestra plays what the conductor decides...just like you have people that work for you and will do what you decide. And the people that work for you are more than capable of doing the things that I will outline in this book.

In respect of time, I won't give you or your staff a bunch of theory either. If you're anything like me, one of the things that you hate is reading a book that has a lot of theory in it before you get to the real meat of what needs to be done. From my point of view, if the author has written a book then they obviously know what they're talking about and you don't need the theory behind it. You don't need the why...you just need the how and the what. So that's what this book is going to focus on...the how and the what with very little theory. I'll give you a step-by-step plan, including the "how" and the "what," to work with.

Some work required

Now, I have to be honest with you doctor and let you know that you're going to have to do a little bit of work here up front. You're going to have to create the musical masterpiece that everybody else is going to play, that everybody else is going to work with. And that's something that only you can do.

So let's jump right into that now so you can get it out of the way, pass this book on to one of your staff members, and get back to taking care of your patients.

4

Chapter 2

ULTIMATE LIFESTYLE TARGET

It's ironic that the very first thing I'm going to ask you to do is to decide on what the end looks like. You've probably heard it before but what we need to do is begin with the end in mind. This is because the "end" is the basis for everything that we're going to do and everything that we're going to be working on. And the way to do this is to go through an exercise that I call the Ultimate Lifestyle Target (ULT) - something I borrowed from one of the greatest marketing minds out there, Frank Kern.

You'll see an example of the Ultimate Lifestyle Target exercise on page 11 but really quickly I'll walk you through what it entails. What you're going to do is figure out how much money you need for all of the "areas" of your life so that you can determine what your yearly income needs to be. And the reason it's called the "Ultimate Lifestyle Target" is because this is where you're going to list all of the things that you want to have in life. It's kind of like a dream machine, if you will, where you're putting down all of your biggest fantasies, fantasies that can be achieved. This is not an exercise where you list out what your current actual expenses are. This is about reaching for the stars! If you really want a Lamborghini™, write it down. Don't worry about how you are going to get it at this point – that part comes later.

Let's charter a private jet to Bora Bora

So there are actually two columns on the list you'll need to fill in. One is the yearly cost and the other is just going to be dividing that number by 12 to figure out how much the item costs monthly. And this list is going to have things like:

- how much your dream home costs...
- how much your dream car costs...
- how much any type of hobbies you have cost...such as flying lessons, boating lessons, gym memberships, jet rentals, playing Pebble Beach every quarter, etc.
- how much your luxury vacations cost...

- how much it would cost, for example, if you wanted to have a personal chef, nanny, housekeeper, gardener, etc.
- how much your fine dining experiences cost...
- how much your trips to the symphony and trips to amusement parks cost...
- how much every day things like your groceries and your random bills cost...
- how much your Christmases cost and how much you want to spend on birthday celebrations...
- how much you want to spend if you have children that are going to go to college...

...and it's going to list how much things are going to cost if you would like to give monetary gifts, let's say, to your parents or to kids or to other relatives that you may have. It's also going to have your retirement and investments in there.

So the key to this is to list out all of the things that you spend money on, as well as all the things that you want to be spending money on, and figure out how much those items cost on a yearly basis. Then break that figure down to find out how much that is on a monthly basis. And you'll see an example on page 11.

Now, the point of this is to figure out how much money, on a monthly basis, you need to be generating from your practice in order to live this ULT and you'll see that it really isn't that much money on a monthly basis when you break it down like this. The problem that I see with most practices is that the doctors don't know how much money they are really – *ideally* – trying to make. They know how much money they would like to make in order to pay their overhead but they really don't have a clear idea of exactly how much money they need to make in their practice in order to live well and meet their ULT...and that's exactly what this exercise helps you do.

So take just a few minutes to fill it out and you'll see some examples here on page 11 that will give you an idea of how much things cost. I live in San Diego, California (things here are much more expensive than they are in other parts of the country) so you may need to adjust these numbers accordingly based on where you live. So go ahead and take maybe 15 minutes at the most to fill this in...and I don't even think that it's going to take 15 minutes...so go ahead and do this exercise now.

[I recommend that you do one of two things...1) do the exercise in this book and be sure to rip the page out afterwards...and don't worry, there's nothing on the back or 2) do it on a separate sheet of paper because you're going to be giving this book to your staff members and you don't want them to see how much money you're actually going to be making when you start doing some of the recommendations in this book. So just take out a separate sheet of paper and fill this information in on that sheet of paper which will leave this book clean for when you give it to other members of your staff.]

Pull out the stops!

One last thing I have to stress here is that I don't want you holding back. This is your Ultimate Lifestyle Target...not your Just Scraping by Target. So you need to shoot for the moon AND shoot for the stars! If you want a 80 foot yacht, write down "80' yacht." If you want to take your family across the country in a private jet, write down "private jet vacations." This is about you and what you really want for yourself and your life - not what you think is realistic or not what you think is possible. The only way that we're going to get you what you want is for you to be clear on exactly what it is that you want. Then we determine how much it costs and what revenue needs to be generated from your practice in order to get there.

ULTIMATE LIFESTYLE TARGET (ULT) - *Example*

Today's Date:_____	Yearly cost	Monthly cost
Oceanview Home	$2,000,000	$16,000
Aston Martin	$125,000	$1,875
Golfing	$5,000	$417
Exotic vacations, 4 per yr.	$60,000	$5,000
Personal chef	$45,000	$3,750
Housekeeper	$25,000	$2,083
Fine dining	$5,000	$417
Groceries	$15,000	$1,250
College	$50,000	$4,167
Practice Overhead[1]	$250,000	$20,833
Total monthly cost of ULT		**$55,792**

[1]Later in the book, we'll discuss ways that you can drastically reduce this figure.

ULTIMATE LIFESTYLE TARGET (ULT) - Exercise

Today's Date_____	Yearly cost	Monthly cost
_____	$_____	$_____
_____	$_____	$_____
_____	$_____	$_____
_____	$_____	$_____
_____	$_____	$_____
_____	$_____	$_____
_____	$_____	$_____
_____	$_____	$_____
_____	$_____	$_____
_____	$_____	$_____
_____	$_____	$_____
_____	$_____	$_____
_____	$_____	$_____
_____	$_____	$_____

Item	Yearly cost	Monthly cost
_____	$_____	$_____
_____	$_____	$_____
_____	$_____	$_____
_____	$_____	$_____
_____	$_____	$_____
_____	$_____	$_____
_____	$_____	$_____
_____	$_____	$_____
_____	$_____	$_____
Total monthly cost of ULT		**$_____**

[Estimate $8,000/month for each $1 million worth of home; $1,500/month for each $100,000 worth of car. FYI, to charter a private jet across the country costs $50,000.]

Now that you've done this, let's take a look at the number from the example: $55,792. Just for the sake of it being a round figure, let's go with a ULT of $56,000. $56,000 per month is what you need to live off of if you're trying to reach your Ultimate Lifestyle Target. Now like I said earlier, depending on where you live, this number may be higher or lower. This figure also depends on what items make up your actual ultimate lifestyle but just for the sake of numbers, let's work with $56,000 per month as your Ultimate Lifestyle Target.

Stop being burned out

Now the next step in this process is for you to figure out how much you really want to work. Since we're talking about your ultimate lifestyle we need to figure out how many hours per day you want to work that will allow you to live your ultimate lifestyle. So for some doctors, you may only want to work 40 hours a week (and I say *only* with tongue-in-cheek). For others, you may only want to work 30 hours per week. I know doctors that work four-day work weeks every week and then take every fourth week off. So what that means is a three day weekend every week and a week's vacation every month. Pretty nice!

So what you need to do now is fill in this information below. It's a single question: how many hours do you want to work per day or per week in order to live your ultimate lifestyle? And there's no right answer here...this is what you want and no one is going to see it but you. And whatever you do, please don't feel guilty or feel bad about only wanting to work 20 hours per week for example. This is your life and your ultimate lifestyle and what we're going for here is what's best for YOU!

How many hours do you want to work:

Per day? _____ Per week?_____

So from here, we need to decide how many days you want to work per week or per month. You may only want to work Monday's, Wednesday's, and Friday's for example. Or like I gave in the previous example, you may only want to work Monday's, Tuesday's, Wednesday's, and Thursday's for three weeks of the month and take the entire last week off. Or you may want to work on Saturday's...it's up to you. You just need to decide, based on your ultimate lifestyle and what ultimately would make you happy, how many days per week you want to work. And keep in mind that it doesn't have to be full days – so it could be Monday's, Tuesday's,

Wednesday's, half day Thursday's, and Fridays off. We're just trying to get an idea here of roughly how many days per week you want to work. For our example, let's use four days per week.

How many days do you want to work:

Per week? _____ Per month?_____

Now we need to take the number of hours you want to work per week (and since this is the ultimate lifestyle, we're going with 30 hours per week) and divide that by the number of days you want to work per week - which is four days from this example. So we're dividing 30 hours per week by four days which gives us 7.5 hours per day. Keep in mind that this is 7.5 hours per day if you decided to divide the hours evenly over the four days...which does not have to be the case.

Now you need to decide how much time you want to spend per patient in order to give them the kind of care that you want them to receive. If you can provide the kind of care that you want to give your patients in 30 minutes then, according to our example, you have 15 open units per day. If your desire is to spend an hour with the patient, and this is the amount of time you feel they need in order to best care for them, from the example you have 7.5 open units.

How much time do you want to spend per patient?

_____

The goal of this exercise is to put you in charge, to help you decide what you want to do. It makes you the conductor of the symphony. You're being proactive as opposed to reacting to what the insurance company decides you should be reimbursed. Reacting is bad because what it results in is you trying to cram as many patients as possible into your practice and into your schedule on a daily basis in order to meet your overhead.

At this point we know how much money you need to make in order to meet your Ultimate Lifestyle Target. We know this monthly (and therefore yearly). We also know how many hours you want to work per week, how many days you want to work per week, how many open units you have per week, and how much time you want to spend per patient.

Now that you have this information, you know what you are aiming for...you know the goal.

Now let's talk about some ways to get you what you want.

[**Note:** If you want to cut "straight to the chase," I recommend you jump to Chapter 6 and read it carefully. Be sure to pay particularly close attention to the "light bulb" moment on page 66.]

Chapter 3

ATTRACTING PATIENTS

It's important to remember that you have the right to *only* work with the kinds of patients you love to treat. Just because you're a doctor doesn't mean you have to take every patient that walks through your door. Now, I know in the past you may have done this because your reimbursements have been declining and you've been trying to get as many patients as possible. But just know that this doesn't **have** to be the case. Remember, you're the doctor and you're in control!

Let's get rid of some of those cobwebs

Now what I want you to do is think back through your medical career and think about the patients that have really made you wake up and come alive, the patients that you've really loved treating...

- Who are these patients?
- What do they look like?
- Are they male or female?
- Are they from a certain socio-economic background?
- Do they have a certain set of characteristics that you love?
- Do they have a disease process that you're really intrigued about?

If you take a look back at these groups of patients that you've enjoyed treating in the past, you'll notice that there is something in common about them...something that you love. It's something that makes you come alive - and those are the exact patients that you should be treating now!

Describe your ideal patient based on the criteria above:

_____

_____

_____

_____

_____

Since we've already determined how many open units you have in your schedule to see patients, it really makes sense that you should fill those open unit slots with the patients that you love treating. So let's talk about what you can do, where you can find, and how you can attract your ideal patients.

Your ideal patients are right under your nose

There are basically two places to find new patients...and I know you may be thinking it sounds crazy to be looking for new patients when you have plenty of patients now (actually too many patients)...but what we're trying to do is replace the patients that you don't enjoy treating with the type of patients that you do enjoy treating.

Two places where you can find patients are: 1) online and 2) offline. Let's talk about the online options first. Doctors who are looking for patients online are successfully using Google Adwords™ and Microsoft AdCenter™ (Yahoo!™ and Bing™), which is "pay-per-click" (abbreviated PPC), to find new patients. PPC is when you set up an ad that shows up in the search results of Google™ or Yahoo!™ and you only get charged (per click) when someone clicks on one of your ads.

One of the fancy words we use in healthcare marketing is "avatar." And basically an avatar is nothing more than a patient profile. It's the patient that you described earlier or that you thought of earlier when you were envisioning your ideal patient. An avatar looks a certain way, has certain interests, is from a certain age group and certain sex, and may or may not have similar interests to yours. This is what you would call an online profile and these patients are very easy to identify online.

The patients that fit your exact patient profile are searching for certain things online. They turn on the computer, they go to Google™ or Yahoo!™, and they type in certain keywords. And when they type these keywords in, Google™ and Yahoo!™ show them ads for practices like yours who are advertising for those keywords. Google Adwords™ and Microsoft AdCenter™ are very clever because the ads are shown over on the right-hand side of the search results and the advertiser, which is you in this situation, is only charged if someone (a prospective patient) clicks on your ad. And when they click on your ad, they're taken to your website. Once you can identify the keyword phrases that your target patient is looking for, it's very easy to go to Google

AdWords™ and/or Microsoft AdCenter™, set up a simple advertising campaign, and start targeting those patients.

[You will find step-by-step instructions in the Tutorials section of this book on setting up a Google AdWords™ account, a Microsoft AdCenter™ account, and posting your first ad. You will find this in Chapter 12.]

What's all the hype about Social Media?

Another even more targeted option is to use Facebook™. Facebook™ has become the juggernaut of social media platforms and the beauty of what they can do is mind boggling. I'm sure you've heard a lot about what Facebook™ can do and how you should be using Facebook™. You've probably heard that you need a fan page, you need a profile page, and all these different things...but the real power behind Facebook™ is in its advertising platform. Whether you know it or not, whether you like it or not, Facebook™ is gathering information about all of its users and it has hundreds of millions of them. And what it does with this information that it gathers about its users is use that information to serve up very targeted advertising... advertising that is very specific to that individual. And in this situation, when I say "individual" think patients.

Here's what Facebook™ does...when you as a user register and fill out your profile page, Facebook™ has software that crawls through the profile and figures out any and all information about you that they can use to serve you very targeted ads. For example, if you listed your favorite book is a Tom Clancy book, they know that you like action, adventure, spy novels, etc. Facebook™ typically knows whether you're male or female, they know what age group you're in, they know what school you went to, they know what associations you belong to, they know what you typically like and don't like, they know so much information about you it's amazing. And this is a great opportunity as an advertiser because you can go into Facebook™, set up an advertising campaign that shows only to people who have certain key words in their profile.

So for example, if there is a Facebook™ user (also known as a potential new patient) that has the word "diabetes" in their profile, you can advertise strictly to them (and anyone else with "diabetes" in their profile). Not only that, but you can advertise just to men (for example) who live within a certain radius or geographic location, who are between the ages of 25 and 35 for example, that like Tom Clancy books...and how ever more specific you want to be. Now this ad may not show to that many people, but what you do know is that the people that it is shown to are very, very targeted and with the right message they are very likely to click on your ad and/or come into your practice.

So what you would do is figure out your ideal patient profile and create an ad that is specifically targeted to other individuals that would fit that profile. You'd also make sure that it is within your target geographic location and write a compelling ad that would get them to call you or stop by your practice for an initial office visit. Facebook™ is probably the most powerful advertising platform on the planet...or at least in the online world.

[You will find step-by-step instructions in the Tutorials section of this book on setting up a Facebook™ business Fan page and posting your first targeted Facebook™ ad. You will find this in Chapter 12.]

Twitter™ and Tweets...

Another online option is Twitter™. And while Twitter™ is not widely used to attract the kinds of patients that you may be looking for, it is being used out there and it is worth knowing about. If you're not familiar with Twitter™, it's an online platform where you have a certain number of characters (140) that you can use to "tweet." And "tweeting" is simply sending out short messages about anything that you want to send out a message about. You could tell the world that you are eating breakfast or that you're going to watch a softball game or that you just saw the most beautiful sunset or whatever suits your fancy. The only people who receive these tweets are people that are following you. So Twitter™ is an excellent way of building a relationship especially considering the fact that nowadays people are craving closer relationships with others...especially with their doctors.

[You will find step-by-step instructions in the Tutorials section of this book on setting up a Twitter™ account and making your first tweet. You will find this in Chapter 12.]

Let's get professional

An additional online option used to attract the kind of patients that you might be looking for is LinkedIn™. LinkedIn™ is an online network of professionals and the users are usually grouped by their area of expertise. This is a great place to attract the kind of patients you're looking for if the kind of patients you're looking for are professionals. The other great thing about LinkedIn™ is that you can use it to let other doctors know about the type of patients that you are interested in and use it to get increased referrals from them. We'll talk about referrals later on in this book.

[You will find step-by-step instructions in the Tutorials section of this book on setting up a LinkedIn™ account and posting your first ad. You will find this in Chapter 12.]

The old-fashioned way...

Now let's talk about the various offline ways you can use to attract the kinds of patients that you're looking for. One way is to use something called a direct mail campaign. A direct mail campaign is when you use some sort of letter, postcard, or other piece that's mailed through the post office/UPS™/FedEx™, etc. The direct mail approach is very effective because it is delivered directly to the mailbox of your prospective patients. You don't have to worry about it going to a spam folder, not being delivered, or not being opened because 99% of everyone out there, when they receive a letter in the mail (if it doesn't look like junk), they open it. The beauty of direct mail is that it can be very targeted as well. Depending on the things your ideal patient buys, the magazines they subscribe to, which credit cards they have, the neighborhoods they live in...all of this information is used to create a consumer (in your case "patient") profile which is easy to sort and segment...and therefore target.

Inside the letter, or on the postcard, you can include information about your practice, a brochure that highlights your services, or any other information that you think your prospective patients might be interested in. Many private practices find that this is an excellent way to recruit new patients.

An additional way many private practices are using to attract new patients is through hiring a marketing company, a PR company, or through hiring a practice management consultant that specializes in acquiring new patients. This can often be an excellent way to get new patients because these companies specialize in this sort of thing and they have been perfecting their technique for many years.

The most important thing to remember is that it all starts with a very clear patient profile. Once you have determined your ideal patient, and have figured out their exact profile, you can use that information for your Google™ ads, for your Facebook™ ads, for your LinkedIn™ ads, for your direct mail pieces and to inform the marketing company, PR company, or practice management consultant about the type of patients you're looking for.

If these things are things you don't see yourself doing – because you don't have the time or you don't want to – give me a call and we'll see if I can help. This is the stuff I love doing and I might be able to do it for you. Of course, there's no charge for us talking or for me coming up with some ideas that will help you.

Promise: *You won't get any sales pitch or pressure from me of any kind...ever!* I can be reached at 858.255.1612 or by email at scartwright@ehealthpriority.com.

Chapter 4

CAPTURING POTENTIAL NEW PATIENT INFORMATION

This is one of the areas I most often see missed in private practices. As a savvy practice owner, you go through all the trouble of attracting patients and getting the new potential patients to your website, but when they're there you need to have an incentive and a method for these potential new patients to leave their names and email addresses. It doesn't do much good for potential new patients to come to your website...but not be interested in coming to see you as a patient right now...and you don't have a way to get back in touch with them to follow up. It's very crucial that you put something on your website that allows you to capture contact information that you can use to get in touch with that potential new patient at a later date.

Healthcare Marketing 101

In marketing terms, the "capture" method is called an "opt-in" box or form. It's a place where website visitors (patients) are asked and incentivized to leave their contact details. Now the easiest way to get a potential new patient to leave their contact information is by using something called a "lead magnet." A lead magnet is also called an "ethical bribe" and it's used to get a potential new patient's name and email address by offering them something of value...but offering it to them for free.

Some examples of lead magnets are:

- Free reports
- DVDs , audio CDs, etc.
- Health checklists
- Free consultations
- Gym memberships
- Mailed health kits, etc.

So when someone comes to your website, one of the first things they see is a free offer for a health consultation and it would say something like *"...for your free 30 minute health consultation, please leave your name and email address below so that we can contact you..."*

Now, if you've taken the time to sit down and think about your ideal patient profile, you'll know the exact type of thing that would get them motivated enough to leave their name and their email address and coming up with the lead magnet should be a piece of cake. The key to this working is that the offer should be something that's very enticing to the potential new patient and something that would make them give you the contact information that you're looking for.

Once a potential new patient leaves their contact information (name, email address, and whatever else you would like to collect), you can use an online program such as Aweber™ (www.aweber.com) or Infusionsoft™ (www.infusionsoft.com) that will collect the information in a database and allow you to email them (collectively as a group) or call them to follow up.

You can also use this approach with potential new patients that call in to your office. From time to time, I put on my *mystery shopper* hat and I call in to a doctor's office just to see how they operate. And what I'll do is I'll ask for the price for a new patient consultation and typically the receptionist will give me the information...I'll say thank you very much, and she'll say bye and hang up. I'm always amazed what a missed opportunity this is for the receptionist (and the practice) but I suppose it's not her fault...she has just never been taught or trained to be better.

When I point it out to you like this, I bet you can see the problem. The receptionist didn't ask me for my contact information by offering me something of value. This would be a great opportunity for the receptionist to say we would like to mail you out a free health checklist or can we have your name and email address so that we can send you a coupon for a free health screenings or free blood sugar test or any variety of things.

You are leaving money on the table

By adopting an ACTIVE potential new patient contact information capturing protocol (that's a mouthful!), your practice would get the contact information for many of the potential new patients that call in and you can use this information to follow up with them at a later date...when it may be a better time for the new patient to come into the practice.

You have to understand that just because someone is not ready to join your practice right now doesn't mean that they won't be ready to join your practice tomorrow or next week or next month. It's important for you to be able to contact that person at a later date and follow up with them to make sure that when they are ready to join a practice, your practice is the first practice that they think of. And the way to do this, to be sure to be "top of mind" when your potential new patient is ready to join a practice, is what we're going to discuss next.

Chapter 5

NURTURING POTENTIAL NEW PATIENTS

The importance of this next step in the process cannot be over emphasized...and you'd be very surprised at how many private practices are not doing this. You've gone through the trouble of attracting potential new patients through online methods, such as Google™, Yahoo!™, Facebook™, etc., and offline through direct mail. You've also set up your website and trained your receptionist so that you can get potential new patient contact information through your very targeted lead magnet. You've offered something of value, such as a free report, DVD, coupon, etc. to get the contact information and now you need to use that contact information in order to nurture your potential new patients.

The stages of decision-making

Now this is important because of the way we, as consumers, make our buying decisions. In the first stage, we are in "thinking mode." So let's say that you're looking for a new carpet cleaner...One day you come home and you start to notice the state of your carpets. You realize that your carpets are dirty and that you need to get them cleaned.

After you've gone through the process of just thinking about it, you move on to the stage of actively researching your options. This looks like looking for carpet cleaners on the internet or perhaps asking friends for some recommendations of good carpet cleaners that they've used.

Once you've gone through your research phase, you make your decision. This decision is based on price or convenience or credibility of the carpet cleaning company. Once you've made your decision, you contact the carpet cleaning company and schedule them to come in and perform the services.

Now this is basically the same process that your potential new patients go through. They move from thinking that they need to find a doctor (unless we're talking about an urgent care situation...which isn't the case most of the time), to research-mode to decision-mode. When they're searching on the internet and call your office to find out about what types of insurance you accept, your practice hours, what their out-of-pocket is going to be, how much is the deductible or copayment, etc. your potential new patients are in research-mode. They're not quite ready to make a decision and you want to position yourself so that you're top of mind when they do decide to make that decision. This is where the nurturing process comes in.

Nurture, nurture...and more nurture...

There are several different ways to nurture your potential new patients. Let's talk about a few of the main ones. One of the most popular options you have for new patient follow-up is an automated email series. An automated email series allows you to write and upload a series of short emails - there could be 3, 5, 7...however many of them that you like - and those emails are delivered automatically over a set period of time and at whatever interval you choose.

So for example, you would designate the first email to be sent one day later (the day after they've left their email address), the second email would go out 3 days later, the third email would go out 6 days later, and so forth.

Now keep in mind that the number of emails and the frequency at which they are delivered is all up to you. One thing you need to know, however, is that you cannot send too many emails. Especially if those emails contain great content and information that your prospective new patients would find valuable and interesting. And because you know the profile of these potential new patients, you know exactly the kind of information that they would be interested in.

Fortunately for you, and for your staff, all of these emails are sent out automatically and the process is initiated as soon as your potential new patient opts-in. So basically, when your potential new patient puts in their name and email address on your website (to get your lead magnet), this automatically adds them into the email responder series and they start to get the emails automatically. If a potential new patient calls in, your receptionist would get your potential new patient's contact information, and then manually add them to the email responder series. This is a very simple process. This way, you stay top of mind with your potential new patients by having regular emails from you in their inbox. These emails always have helpful information which greatly increases the chances of them calling you once they have made their decision.

Be careful...

Very few practices are doing this and you'll be amazed at the response you'll get when you start doing this. The key to this working well is that you have to target your ideal potential new patients from the very beginning. This follow-up and nurture process doesn't discriminate. It nurtures any potential new patient that comes into the system. So it will attract patients that you don't want to see as easily as it will attract patients that you do want to see. For this reason it's vitally important that you only attract and nurture your ideal potential patient...and you do this by targeting them accordingly at the very beginning.

There are several email responder programs out there to choose from. There are companies such as Aweber™ (www.aweber.com) & Mail Chimp™ (www.mailchimp.com) that are very inexpensive and there are higher-end products, such as Infusionsoft™ (www.infusionsoft.com), that are much more robust and do a lot more things.

Disconnect so you can re-connect...

Another popular option for nurturing potential new patients is to use direct mail. We talked about direct mail a little earlier in this book and it's the same concept. You'll be mailing out letters, postcards, bulky mail pieces, etc...anything that you would like to send that would keep you top of mind with your potential new patients.

There are companies out there that specialize in very inexpensive handwritten letters that you can use. The letters are written on yellow, lined paper and look like they have come personally from you. They are actually hand-written...you just don't have to sit there and write them out. You can find out more information about handwritten letters by contacting James Cappelmann at www.upperhandmarketing.com. Be sure to tell him I told you to call and he'll take good care of you!

There are other online software programs that generate postcards and mail them out on your behalf. You simply set up an account, have someone input the contact information, pick out the appropriate greeting card or postcard, and it automatically sends it out with your personalized message. You can find out more information about sending greeting cards at www.sendoutcards.com/112936.

Additionally, you could send out coupons, invitations to open houses, invitations to come in and meet you and your staff, etc. There's no end to the possible options of direct mail. And again...so few practices are doing this that you'll be a standout. Just imagine how impressed you would be if you had contacted a potential new carpet cleaner to get a quote and after you hung up with them a couple of days later you received a postcard or handwritten letter in the mail from the carpet cleaning company. The postcard would be a coupon for 50% off your first carpet cleaning or the handwritten letter would be used to introduce the owner of the carpet cleaning company, let you know how long they've been in business, and offer you a special discount for becoming a new client of theirs. I think it's safe to say that you would be quite impressed and that you would most likely use their services as opposed to any of the other services from carpet cleaners you had contacted that did not contact you back.

Another way to nurture potential new patients is by going "old school" and picking up the telephone and making a phone call. In this day and age we get so wrapped up with technology and all the things that technology will do for you but sometimes the old-fashioned approach is the best approach.

Let's say a potential new patient calls in inquiring about the insurance that you accept and your receptionist offers her a free report on how to select the best family medicine doctor ...and she takes your receptionist up on her offer. In order to get the free special report she leaves her contact information, which includes a phone number, with your receptionist. A couple of days later, your receptionist calls her and asks her if she has any further questions and if there's anything that she can do to help with her decision process.

We're not talking about a hard sale or anything like that. We're just talking about calling and genuinely offering to be of assistance to someone who's trying to make a decision. Perhaps your office is not the best fit for this potential new patient and your receptionist could refer them to some other doctor that you know of that you think would be a better fit. Anything is possible when your staff is truly trying to be helpful.

During the phone call, your receptionist could ask if the potential new patient would be interested in coming in for a private tour of the office, or sitting down to "interview" the doctor, or taking part in a free health assessment. The sky really is the limit here on what you can offer and never underestimate how powerful a simple phone call can be. Potential new patients, more than anything else, are looking to connect with their doctor (and the staff in their doctor's office) and this phone call is a nice personal touch and a way to show your potential new patient that you care and that your practice's main goal is to be helpful.

Let's not get crazy here!

If you're feeling really ambitious, you can do a mix of old-school and new school. What I'm referring to is using automated outbound telephone calls to place the calls for you. There are companies out there that specialize in placing automated outbound telephone calls. So what happens is you record a pre-recorded message, upload it to their system, and it automatically sends out the pre-recorded message to everyone who you tell it to send it to.

So your receptionist would input the phone number(s) and the system would send the pre-recorded message out to your potential new patients at a predetermined time. In the phone call, you would introduce yourself, tell a little bit about your medical training, tell them about your area of specialty, and anything else you think they may want to know. This gives your potential new patients a chance to get to know you a little bit better without requiring you or your receptionist to make the outbound calls. You can find out more information about sending pre-recorded telephone messages at www.voiceshot.com.

What really works well however, is a combination of personal outbound phone calls and automated outbound phone calls. Your receptionist (or whoever you designated) would make the *personal* outbound phone call and answer any questions that your potential new patients may have and your pre-recorded voice message would be on the *automated* outbound phone calls.

Whatever you do, be sure to incorporate some form of new patient nurturing into your process whether it be email, direct mail, or phone calls.

Chapter 6

MAKING MORE MONEY

We're now getting to the real meat and potatoes...the reason you bought this book – to make more money!

Now, making more money may not be what motivates you. What probably motivates you is taking care of patients and helping people – that's what really motivates you...I mean, that's why you became a doctor right?

Just think about how much easier it would be to take care patients if you weren't:

- Always worried about money
- Trying to see as many patients as possible in a single day

- Worried about your declining insurance reimbursements
- Concerned about what the government was going to do next

What if you didn't have to worry about any of that and you could just focus on seeing patients and taking better care of those patients...wouldn't that be great?

The decision is yours...

We always come to a fork in the road...a moment of decision. You're going to have to decide if you want to make more money by working harder OR if you want to make more money by working smarter.

Up until this point in the book we've mostly been focused on working harder. I've told you what you need to do in order to attract more new potential patients, how to get those new potential patients' contact information, and how to nurture them. And hopefully when you're doing these things and going through the process I outlined, you're only attracting and capturing the contact information and nurturing your ideal potential patient. It doesn't make much sense to go through this process and attract the patients that you don't want to work with. Now this method, as I mentioned earlier, is working harder. You would be trying to get more patients in order to make more money. [Caveat: the attract-capture-nurture process can be used to work *smarter* as well.]

Due to the fact that there are a set number of hours in the day, and a set number of hours that you're available to see patients, there are only two ways to make more money in your private practice. You can either see more patients during your available hours or you can increase the value (to you) of the patients you are currently seeing...which is just another way of saying make more money per patient.

Let's do a little math

You see...I like to keep things simple. Not necessarily so much for you...but for me. I've found it much easier to understand and explain things when they are simple and in black-and-white terms. If you have 10 hours a day to see patients and you want to make more money, you can either see more patients during those 10 hours or you can charge more money to the patients that you're already seeing during those 10 hours. These are the only two options. One of them is working harder and the other is working smarter.

Now, I want you to look back at the numbers you came up with when you were doing your ideal number of hours worked per day/week exercise, your ideal number of days worked per week/month exercise, and the ideal amount of time you wanted to spend with each patient exercise. [From Chapter 2] Considering those numbers, only YOU can decide if working harder is something that fits in with your ultimate ideal lifestyle.

The HARSH reality...

If you want to double your practice income, you're going to need to see twice as many patients as you are currently seeing while continuing to work the number of hours that you are currently working. [Side note: you will probably need to see **more** than double the current number of patients that you're seeing (AND increase the number of hours you are working) in order to double your income due to the continual decrease in insurance reimbursements.] If you want to triple your practice income, you're going to need to see three times as many patients... I think you get the picture.

Question for you...Can you reach your Ultimate Lifestyle Target, which will allow you to lead your ideal ultimate lifestyle, by working harder? Yes / No [circle one]

If you answered YES, keep reading because from this point on, we're going to be talking about working smarter (even if you still plan on working harder up to this point...meaning doing all the things we talked about in Chapters 1 through 5)....

If you answered NO, keep reading...

The SOLUTION...

The alternative to working harder (seeing more patients per hour) is to work smarter by making more money per patient. Remember that the goal here is to keep you in charge, make you the conductor of the symphony, and keep you from becoming an employee of the hospital. You deserve to get paid what you're worth, not what the government or insurers say you'll be paid!

There are several ways to do this - to work smarter not harder. Let's talk about one that is increasing in popularity by the day (especially considering the changes that are happening in the field of medicine): developing a direct financial relationship with your patients, a.k.a. Concierge Medicine.

These days, concierge medicine is going by a lot of different names – exclusive practice (as opposed to "private practice"), personalized medicine, private medicine, celebrity medicine, direct care, direct primary care, private doctors, VIP care, etc. In the past, there was a negative connotation to the concept of concierge medicine (which I will refer to as "direct care" moving forward). It was thought to be elitist and it was not strongly embraced by the medical community. Today, however, we are in a new era in medicine and direct care is becoming widely accepted as a viable alternative to traditional private practice.

Why it may be right FOR YOU

Practicing a direct care model allows you to:

- See fewer patients and spend more time with them (getting to know them better)

...which means you get to **take better care** of them!

- Interact with your patients in person, by phone, by email, or on the internet

...which means you get to really feel like you are doing your job as a doctor again!

- **Make more money**

...which means you will *finally* get paid what you are worth!

- Spend more time with your family and do the things you love

...which means you get to be with your spouse/ significant other, see your kids grow up, and take more time off!

- Stop playing by Medicare and the insurance companies' rules

...which means YOU get to call the shots in your practice and you won't have to worry about any upcoming reimbursement cuts!

- Spend less time on administrative and non patient-related issues

...which means you get to keep the kinds of notes you want, cut out all the red tape, and get rid of the unnecessary staff and the companies that will no longer be needed – **decreasing your overhead!**

...all through a financial relationship that you have directly with your patients. Ultimately, this model allows you to, in essence, cutout out the middleman (the insurance company) and allows you to practice medicine on your own terms. It also significantly decreases your overhead and the administrative burden of practicing medicine because you are no longer billing the insurance companies (if you do decide to convert to the "pure model" – discussed later) and you are not worried about CPT codes and billing codes and making sure you are maintaining the proper medical record documentation, etc.

Why it's right for YOUR PATIENTS

Practicing a direct care model *also* allows your patients to have:

- **Overall better health** (studies have shown that patients with a direct financial relationship with their doctor experience better health outcomes and make less trips to the hospital).
- Same day or next day appointments

- A more personal and intimate relationship with you
- A better quality of life due to preventative medicine practices (which includes nutrition counseling)

Your options

The beauty of today's direct care model is just that...that it is a model. It is a framework in which you can set up your practice any way you choose. You have the choice of setting up a pure direct care practice where all of your patients are members. In this model, you go through a conversion process where you will invite your current patients to become members of your new practice. The pros of this model are:

1. You'll be seeing less patients and therefore able to spend the more quality time per patient
2. You won't be filling out any insurance paperwork
3. You won't have to pay for a billing or coding specialist
4. You'll be working less hours and able to take more time off

The cons of this model are:

1. It's a riskier proposition because you must go through a conversion process and you may not get the number of patients that you would like [In Chapter 7 we will discuss a process that can help prevent this from happening]
2. You may be reluctant to turn away patients that you already have ("a bird in the hand" mentality)
3. You may not like the perceived perception that you are a doctor that only cares about money and not about patients

You also have the choice of setting up a "hybrid" direct care practice where you invite your current patients to become members and those that do not become paying members are still able to see you. The pros of this model are:

1. You'll be making more money than you currently are
2. It's less riskier because you don't have to worry about meeting a certain target number of patients
3. You don't have to get rid of any of your current patients
4. You don't have to worry about the negative perceived perception

The cons of this model are:

1. You'll be working just as hard, if not harder, due to the fact that you'll be spending more time with your direct care patients while at the same time seeing the patients that did not convert to direct care patients

2. You'll still be filing billing claims with insurance companies and therefore still have that as an overhead and administrative burden

3. There would be a noticeable and perceived disparity between the service and treatment your direct care patients are receiving versus the service and treatment your regular patients are receiving

One thing to note however, is that in the hybrid model you can decide to NOT accept insurance (meaning you don't file necessary billing information with the insurance company), but you do provide the necessary materials, such as a super bill, for the patients who want to file the claim with their insurance company themselves.

Remember...YOU are the conductor

There are two very important things to keep in mind as you are considering setting up your direct care model. One is that there is no "one-size-fits-all." Every practice is different and what's right for you and your practice may not be right for another practice.

The second is that "the sky is the limit." You can set up your direct care model any way you like. You can make it a hybrid version where your office processes the insurance information, a hybrid version where your office doesn't process the information, you can charge a monthly membership fee to get "access" to you and then maintain your practice the way it is currently set up (meaning continuing billing your patients' insurance), you can charge a monthly fee that covers all of your services, or anything else you can possibly think of. The sky really is the limit!

Likewise, the amount of money you charge per patient - for access to you or for services - is completely up to you. There are direct care doctors out there charging as little as $50 per month per patient all the way up to $4,200 per month for some families...and everything in between! Your choice will be based on what works best for YOU, the healthcare provider, and then you'll just have to clearly explain the value of what you provide and the benefits to your future direct care patients.

You need some help?

If you think the direct care model may be right for you but you don't see yourself setting it up by yourself – because you don't have the time or you don't want to – give me a call and we'll see if I can help. This is the stuff I love doing and I might be able to do everything for you. Of course, there's no charge for us talking or for me coming up with some ideas that will help you.

Promise: *You won't get any sales pitch or pressure from me of any kind...ever!* I can be reached at 858.255.1612 or by email at scartwright@ehealthpriority.com.

What about Medicare?

One commonly asked question is, can I have a direct financial relationship with some patients and see other patients with Medicare. The answer to this question is yes...with one caveat...as long as the services that you provide your direct care patients are services that Medicare does not cover. For example, cosmetic procedures. Or even something more concrete such as preventative or nutritional counseling. So if you pair up an extensive physical with preventative services, such as nutrition counseling – something not covered by Medicare – you are good to go.

You might be wondering...

Let me answer a few other questions that might be on your mind...

What is the average panel size for the average primary care physician?

- 2,300

According to published research, how many patients can a primary care physician reasonably care for?

- 1,620

According to published research, what is the ideal patient panel size?

- Fewer than 1,000 patients

What is the average patient panel size for a direct care practice?

- Between 200 to 600 patients

What is the average time traditional primary care physicians spend with their patients?

- Some reports say 6 to 8 minutes while other reports say 13 to 15 minutes

How much time do direct care doctors spend with their patients?

- Typically 45 minutes to one hour or more

How much does the average direct care, primary care physician charge per year, per patient?

- $1,800 per year ($150 per month)

With an average patient panel of 2,500, if I do it on my own, how many patients can I expect to convert to a direct care model?

- Between 175 to 250 patients

With an average patient panel of 2,500, if I get professional help, how many patients can I expect to convert a direct care model?

- Between 400 to 500 patients.

Now, I want you to look back at the Ultimate Lifestyle Target (ULT) figure you came up with in Chapter 2. For our example, the amount was $56,000 per month.

At $56,000 per month, you would only need 373.33 (we'll round up to 375) patients paying you the national average of $150 per month. **Just 375 patients!**...out of the thousands of patients you currently have on your panel.

At $200 per month, you only need 280 patients and at $250 per month, you only need 224 patients.

You might want to sit down for this but I want you to take your monthly ULT figure and divide it by $150, $200, and $250 - just to give you an idea of how <u>few</u> patients you'll have to convert to reach your ultimate target income level...AND you'll be taking <u>better</u> care of them!

Are you smiling yet? =)

Chapter 7

LAUNCHING YOUR "NEW" PRACTICE

[You should skip this chapter if you haven't decided you want to make more money, see less patients, and practice medicine on your terms using the direct care model.]

Once you have decided to adopt the direct care model, or any variation thereof, one of the most critical parts of the process is the actual conversion itself. And by "conversion" I mean the actual conversion process you go through to convert your current patients into patients who have a direct financial relationship with you. I say this is one of the most critical parts because this conversion process, and the subsequent "new" patients (which are actually your current patients that have a "new" relationship with you) that it generates, will be the foundation for your new practice moving forward. It is vitally essential that you get this part right.

Like a product launch...but BETTER!

In order to successfully convert your practice from a traditional model to a direct care model, you're going to need to go through a process that I call a "New Practice Launch." You're going to want to create a lot of interest, "buzz," and excitement about what you're doing and make your patients feel like they will be missing out on something very special if they are not a part of it.

To get an idea of what I'm talking about, I want you to think back about some of the successful "product" launches you've seen in the past. Perhaps it was for new restaurant in your area or, even better, think back about the launch of the iPhone™.

If you recall, they created so much hype and buzz around the release of the iPhone™ that you could practically feel it. Every few weeks, before the official release date of the iPhone™, there were leaks of the phone's diagrams. Then someone would "slip" and tell how fast the processor was or how big the screen was. The icing on the cake was when someone high up on the product engineering team "accidentally" left one of the new iPhones™, before it had been released, in a bar near San Francisco. These stories got so much publicity in the news, and were talked about by so many people, that it made people want an iPhone™ who didn't even originally want one. This is the type of excitement that we want to create for your "new" practice. The New Practice Launch is the perfect way to do this.

The simple steps

The New Practice Launch turns what could easily be a mundane process into an event that your patients can't stop talking about...and it keeps it "top of mind." The launch includes a few key steps with specific goals for each step. These steps are:

1. Pre-prelaunch
2. Pre-launch
3. Launch
4. Post-launch

Before we talk about the goals of each one of these steps, let's talk about the *ultimate* goal of your launch. In addition to creating buzz and excitement, the ultimate goal of your New Practice Launch is to convert as many patients as possible (or at least your target number of patients) into patients who have a direct financial relationship with you. In addition to the goal of the launch, you'll need to come up with a "back story," including why you are changing your practice from a traditional practice to a direct care practice, as well as what services you'll be offering in your new practice...and the fee.

By "back story" I mean you'll need to have given some thought to, and be able to clearly articulate, why you're changing things. Your current patients are going to want to know what's going on and more importantly, they're going to want to know why. Change is always difficult [the only thing that *likes* change is a wet baby =)] and your patients are going to instinctively resist change unless you tell them your motivation and the reasons behind why the change is taking place.

You could be converting your practice for many reasons, such as:

- You feel like you'll be able to provide better service
- You want to make sure your current patients always have access to you
- You want to make sure your patients get the time that they deserve

- You want to make sure they stay as healthy as possible
- You don't want to be bogged down with unnecessary administrative paperwork
- You were getting burnt out
- Etc.

...or any combination of the above. What's important is that you and your staff are honest as to the reasons behind the conversion and that everyone on your staff is on the same page when the inevitable questions arise.

Remember...calculate risks and act decisively...

I think it's important to point out at this point that once you decide to convert your practice to a direct care model, you have to know that the decision has been made. You and your staff cannot come across as wishy-washy or "iffy" or uncertain about what you're doing. You cannot give the impression that this is not a done deal. Your patients are going to be wondering what to do and they will be looking to you and your staff for leadership and confidence. No one wants to be involved with someone who is unsure of themselves.

Lastly, before we get into the launch steps, you need to come up with exactly what you're offering including:

- What services you'll be providing
- What kind of access your patients will have to you
- What your response time will be
- The time frame for office visits
- Etc.

...and how much you will be charging. Now let's move on to the specific goals of the launch steps.

Pre-prelaunch. The goal of this step is to let your patients know that something BIG is happening and to build early buzz and excitement. This stage is used as a warming process and used to convey your story, including the "why," of the upcoming conversion. It's also used to identify and counter any potential objections that your current patients may have. One great way to execute this step is to use an electronic survey sent out to all your patients. You can use an online service called Survey Monkey™ (www.surveymonkey.com) that will create this electronic survey and collect the responses for you. There is a free version as well as several paid versions of the software - each with different options.

At the beginning of the survey you would let your patients know that something important is happening within your practice and then ask them to answer a few, short survey questions – all designed to give you more insight into exactly what it is that they are looking for. You will then use their responses and their concerns as you move into the next steps.

Pre-launch. The goal of this step is to let your patients know about the conversion, create anticipation, bring the buzz and excitement levels to their peak, reveal all the details, and facilitate an open dialogue, between you and your patients, which includes letting them know how many patients you plan on accepting and what will happen if they "miss the boat." Fear of loss is a powerful motivator and if done correctly, with honesty and integrity, you should have no problem reaching your target number of patients.

The execution of this step is best done through a series of free reports (where you send your patients written information about things they care about), videos (same concept as the free reports except this is recorded in video format as either live-action videos or recorded PowerPoint presentations), and webinars or tele-seminars (live events where you invite your patients to join you as a group on the telephone or on the internet. During these events you present some valuable information and/or do a question-and-answer session.).

These things may seem scary to you right now but I want to assure you that they are easy to do. With technology that currently exists, these daunting tasks are quite easy to pull off. These steps engage your patients while simultaneously educating them. This type of relationship building is exactly what you're looking for as you're building anticipation, buzz and excitement. It also pre-conditions your patients to the excellent service and health education they will receive by entering into a direct financial relationship with you.

Launch. The goal of this step is to "open the doors" and let your new patients in. If everything is done properly in the pre-prelaunch stage and in the pre-launch stage, this will be the easy part. You will have created so much anticipation and excitement, built a stronger personal relationship with your patients, and let them know what the consequences are of missing out, that they will be chomping at the bit to become one of your new patients.

The trick to making this a successful step is to have everything lined up in advance with your payment processor. Don't forget that you're going to be accepting monthly payments (by credit card) for your services. These credit cards will need to be processed every month and you'll need a payment processor that will be able to take care of that for you automatically. There are many services out there that will do this for you and you will need to do a little bit of research to find one that fits your needs. Free online services, such as PayPal™ (www.paypal.com), can be set up to process recurring payments and will only charge you when they process the payment. Other online providers charge a flat monthly fee, plus certain per-transaction fees, and have more robust services.

You may even decide to charge a joining, application, or initial membership fee...which is not unheard of. The main thing to remember here is to have everything set up so that when your new patients are ready to give you money, you have a way to accept the money and a way to automatically sign them up for monthly/quarterly/semi-annually/annually recurring billing.

I typically recommend a 14-day to 21-day New Practice Launch period with the various elements (including emails) spaced 3 to 4 days apart. This can, of course, be changed based on your current situation.

Don't be OVERWHELMED!

If doing a New Practice Launch makes you feel uncomfortable, don't let that stop you. If you feel like you don't have the time or you don't want to be bothered, give me a call and we'll see if I can help. I have done many successful product launches and this is the stuff I love doing. I might be able to do it for you. Of course there's no charge for us talking or for me coming up with some ideas that will help you.

Promise: *You won't get any sales pitch or pressure from me of any kind...ever!* I can be reached at 858.255.1612 or by email at scartwright@ehealthpriority.com.

Post-launch. The goal of this step is to "deliver and satisfy"...which ultimately means taking care of patients. We'll be discussing this topic, at length, in Chapter 9.

Chapter 8

COLLECTING CASH

Collecting the cash is the area where I see most doctors' offices doing pretty good. Your office is probably set up to take credit cards, checks, and even cash, if necessary, and your patients are using these to pay for their co-pays, deductibles, and uncovered procedures. Additionally, you probably have someone that's responsible for the billing in your practice or you outsource it to a billing company.

You may not have thought of...

If you are doing all of your billing in-house, you might want to consider a couple options to increase your practice revenue.

1. Outsource your billing to a billing company. There are several reputable billing companies out there who do nothing but provide billing services to

private practices. These billing companies are great because the people who work for these companies are experts in billing and their livelihood is based on you getting the most money from the evaluation, management, and procedures you perform in your office.

There are also professional medical billing specialists out there who don't work for private companies but instead work for themselves...typically out of their homes. These billers can often be hired at a fraction of the cost of those working for companies simply because they don't have the same overhead that the companies have and they can pass the savings along to you.

One of the best places to find these types of billers is by doing a simple search on Craigslist in your area. If you've never used Craigslist before, you'll be surprised at the sheer number, and qualifications, of the billing specialists that you'll find. If you can't find a billing specialist by searching on Craigslist in your area, for $25 per category, you can post an open position in your practice and let those looking for a job find and contact you.

2. Hire a company that specializes in revenue management. One thing that I know for sure is that "you don't know what you don't know." And as much as we hate to admit it, there are some things that we just don't know. When it comes to the revenue in your practice, you don't know what money you might be leaving on the table. You may think that everything that you are doing in terms of billing is correct, but in reality, it very well may not be. Or it may be correct but there are things that you are not billing for that you *could* be billing for or things that you are doing that you are under-billing for. There is really no way to know unless you make the decision to get professional help.

If you do a quick Google™ search for "revenue management," "billing and coding specialists," "medical practice billing," "maximize medical practice billing," etc. you'll get a good idea of all the different companies out there, including the consultants, that can help you increase your practice's bottom line.

Now should you decide to go with the "work smarter not harder" direct care model, there are several things you need to consider. One of the most important things to consider is how much money you want to charge per patient – or per family – and what will your patient get for this money. Will they be receiving access to you for this fee (and either you or they will still be billing their insurance) or will your fee include services? And if so, what specific services are covered in this fee?

When adopting a direct care model, this will probably be the area that you struggle with the most. I can tell you now that you're going to have all kinds of conversations with yourself. You'll be wondering...

- How much is too much to charge...and how much is too little?
- If your patients will really be willing to pay for this
- If you're going to ostracize yourself from some of your longtime patients or your colleagues
- If medicine should be boiled down to ability to pay, etc.

All of this "self talk" is healthy, but don't let yourself talk you out of charging what you are truly worth. At the end of the day, you must remember that you are the doctor – the conductor – and you need to be compensated fairly for the role you play in society and in your patients' lives.

What are other doctors charging?

When deciding on your fee, keep in mind that the national average for doctors practicing the direct care model is $150 per patient, per month. Now, I say "keep this in mind" just to give you a reference point. Some doctors are charging as little as $50 per month while others, on the high end, are charging $1250 per month...and everything in between.

A few things you'll want to remember when determining your fee are:

- What are the demographics of your current patient panel?
- What are the demographics of your neighborhood (or the area where you draw your patients from)?
- What is the socio-economic status of your current patient panel?

- What is the socio-economic status around your practice and the neighborhoods you draw from?
- What is the scarcity or saturation level of other doctors in your area?
- What is the perceived need to see a doctor in your area?
- Etc.

Whatever you do, don't sell yourself short! Take a look at your Ultimate Lifestyle Target, fully appreciate the important role you play in your patients' lives, and then set your fee accordingly. And at this point, I'd even go so far as to say that once you've picked your price, add an additional $50 to $100 on top of it and make that your price...and then sit back and be amazed at how many patients will gladly pay it.

And to understand why so many of your patients will gladly pay it, you need to understand what's going through your patients' minds right now. They're constantly being bombarded through the news and through their friends about how many more people, that didn't have insurance before, are now covered by way of Obamacare. We're talking 32 million more people!

They know that there are going to be **long waits** to see a doctor...and your patients don't want to be left out in the cold when it comes to their health care. They will gladly pay you because:

1. They have already established a relationship with you
2. They want to be able to see you in a timely fashion and are concerned about getting squeezed out with all the 32 million people who now have insurance coverage, and
3. They want better access to you, more time with you, and better care from you...especially as they age.

Don't sell yourself short. I'll say that one more time... Do **not** sell yourself short!

Another consideration...

Something else to consider, should you decide to convert to a direct care model, is that you will no longer need help with billing. Whether you're currently using an in-house billing specialist or a billing company, when you are no longer accepting insurance, or reduced insurance, or having your patients file their own claims, you'll no longer need the level of billing support that you currently have. This will be a considerable monthly financial savings.

Your 2 new favorite words: Recurring income

One thing that you'll have to get, however, is a merchant account that allows you to do recurring billing payments. Recurring billing payments are something that happen monthly, like clockwork, without you or your staff having to do anything manually. So for example, should you determine your monthly access fee is $250, your patients would be billed $250 per month, every month, starting on the day they decide to become one of your new direct care patients. Setting this up automatically is important because you don't want to be charging credit cards manually every day.

What this means to you is that you will:

- Get to experience a steady flow of income
- Be able to better manage the finances of your practice,
- Get paid what you are worth
- No longer deal with insurance companies and depend on reimbursements

...and it all happens automatically!

There are many software applications out there that will do this for you – Infusionsoft™ (www.infusionsoft.com) being one of the most robust and capable systems. But starting off, you could use something as simple as PayPal™ that allows you to set up recurring billing for your patients using their credit card information. You simply set up a PayPal™ account (www.paypal.com), set up a product and/or recurring billing amount, input your patient's name and credit card information, and every month the system will bill their credit card and collect the money for you. It doesn't get any better than this!

[You will find step-by-step instructions in the Tutorials section of this book on setting up a PayPal™ account and adding recurring billing. You will find this in Chapter 12.]

Chapter 9

TAKING CARE OF PATIENTS

Now...let's move on to the good stuff! In this chapter we're going to talk about something that I'm sure is near and dear to your heart. It's the reason you went into medicine and the reason you endured years and years of training. I think it's safe to say that you like helping people and, more specifically, you love taking care of patients. And not just taking care of them but you really like seeing them get better.

Providing GREAT care

I'm sure you've realized that one of the things that really helps you take care of your patients, and helps them get better, is learning about them on a personal level. Once you know:

- Their history
- What makes them tick
- What things they are likely to do
- Which recommendations they're not likely to follow
- How things are in their home environment
- Etc.

... it can make your job as a doctor much, much easier.

The problem you know all too well

The problem with the way that you are forced to practice medicine these days is that you're not given the time that you need in order to form these personal relationships with your patients. You're expected to:

- See patients in anywhere from 10 to 15 minutes (in order to make ends meet) which barely gives you enough time for pleasantries let alone getting to know your patients better
- Sort through the details for their visit
- Write any prescriptions that they may need

- Take care of any paperwork that they need filled out (such as leave of absence paperwork)
- Etc.

...not to mention writing your notes!

This being the case, your patients are NOT getting any better and you probably feel you're not doing the best job that you can do (even though I'm sure you're doing the best that you *can* do under the current circumstances). Well, it doesn't have to be this way and the direct care model is at the top of the list of the easiest and best options for you to be able to take better care of your patients (and yourself!).

What you can expect for your patient care

Doctors who have converted to the direct care model report, and studies confirm, that:

- They are able to see patients for 45 minutes to an hour (and sometimes longer)
- They are able to form strong relationships with their patients
- Their patients have better outcomes
- Their job satisfaction is much higher than those doctors who are in traditional private practice.

I'm sure you can see how all of this would be true.

One thing we've already discussed, if you're still hesitant about converting to a pure direct care model, is seeing both direct care patients as well as traditional patients within your existing practice. I won't re-hash the pros and cons of this approach at this point but just know that it's a viable option if you'd like to test the waters or "ease" into the direct care model. [You can find the pros and cons in Chapter 6.]

Showing up is half the battle

Now, whether you decide to stay in traditional private practice or convert to a direct care model – or some form of "hybrid" model – the only way to treat patients and help them get better is to actually have them show up for their appointments. Let's look at and discuss some of the ways that you can increase your chances of having your patients show up for their appointments. Let's work from the most effective to the least effective.

1. Text message reminders

This is easily the most effective way to communicate with your patients and to ensure that they don't miss their upcoming appointments. Studies show that 97% of people with cell phones will read their incoming text messages within 15 minutes of receiving them. 84% of people with cell phones will respond to those incoming text messages within an hour. If used 24 and 48 hours prior to an appointment, text messages can be used as a gentle and convenient reminder about upcoming appointments.

If you do a quick search in Google™ for "text message reminders" or "text message follow-up service," you'll find many affordable options...some of them even free! If you're not currently using text message reminders, I strongly suggest that you start using them as soon as possible. When you do, you'll notice a dramatic decrease in your no-show rate.

2. Live phone call reminders

Actually having someone from your office pick up the telephone and call your patients, reminding them of their appointments, is very effective. There are several automated options out there (which we'll talk about next) but nothing is quite as effective as a good ole telephone call. 24 and 48 hours prior to an appointment, someone from your office should pick up the telephone, call your patients, and not call it a day until they have spoken with each patient on the list. And "spoken with each patient" does not mean leave a message for the patient.

It's very important that your office staff knows that leaving a voicemail is not the same as actually speaking with the patient. The reason is that some messages get lost in the clutter – just like everything else – and once you've actually *spoken* to a patient, they're more likely to keep their appointment or, at a minimum, let you know that they need to cancel the upcoming appointment that they have. This live telephone call can also be used to:

- Answer any last minute questions that your patients may have
- Remind them to bring anything special that they need for their visit
- Take care of anything that would be easy to take care of over the phone.

The challenge with placing live, outbound telephone calls is that they can be very time-consuming. But as I mentioned, nothing beats a live phone call and the personal touch that it lets your office convey.

3. Automated phone call reminders

Automated phone calls to your patients are a good way to remind them about upcoming appointments but they are nowhere near as good as live phone calls. When you have an automated phone call sent, there's no way to make sure that the phone call or voicemail message is actually received by your patient. If anyone else in the household gets the phone call or voicemail message, they may not pass that message on to your patient...which defeats the purpose of this reminder.

Using automated phone call messages may also violate your patient's HIPPA rights if someone other than the intended patient receives the phone call or voicemail message. Automated phone calls also do not allow you to deal with any last minute, real-time issues that come up with pending appointments. The flipside of this is that automated phone calls allow you to use technology to decrease the workload of your staff.

4. Email reminders

Email reminders, while better than nothing, are probably the least effective tool that you can use to remind your patients about upcoming appointments. Approximately 65% of all emails sent are spam...so your patients have grown accustomed to deleting or not looking at most of the emails that come into their inboxes. By using email reminders, you also run the risk of your patients never even seeing your emails because often times the emails are diverted directly to the spam folder. In addition, the email industry today is experiencing about a 35% open rate for health related and medical emails. This means that if your email does get past the spam filter, it only stands at 35% chance of being opened.

The secret to having a great plan in place to decrease your no-show rate is to use 2 or more of the methods mentioned in this chapter when reminding your patients about their upcoming appointments. The more methods you use, the more you increase your chances of having your patients show up for their appointments.

Chapter 10

INCREASING PATIENT VALUE

In order for you to make more money in your practice, while simultaneously maintaining your current patient panel size (or even by seeing less patients), you only really have 2 options:

1. Seeing the patients that you do have MORE OFTEN
2. Increasing the transaction value per patient... meaning, collecting more money per patient, per visit.

We've already discussed collecting (more) money per patient by using the <u>direct care model</u> (assessing an access, membership, or services fee) but there are other ways to increase your current patient value as well.

These include:

1. **Diabetes Management**. Hire a professional or train one of your staff members to provide diabetes management, education, and training to your patients who would benefit from these types of classes. You could develop a 6-, 8-, or 10-week program that your patients would go through (in your office) where they learn everything they need to know about nutrition, medication, exercise, etc. and you could bill their insurance companies or Medicare for providing these services. Depending on how you set up the program, your patients could be billed for going through group training or private training.

Don't forget, pre-diabetes is a subcategory that you can provide training on as well. With approximately 80 million people with pre-diabetes in the United States, your current patient panel is bound to provide you with many patients who could use these types of classes.

2. **Weight-Loss Counseling**. Similar to the concept above, you can provide weight loss counseling to your patients who are currently struggling with keeping their weight under control. Medicare has

incentivized this type of training in doctors' offices by agreeing to reimburse for these services. Your patients must meet certain criteria, such as BMI, specific risk factors, etc. in order to qualify for reimbursement, but once their eligibility has been determined you're able to bill for weight loss counseling as appropriate.

You can also form partnerships and negotiate terms with local gyms and fitness clubs. The thought here is that you make referrals or recommendations to fitness clubs to the patients that would benefit. You could even negotiate with the gyms and fitness clubs to have them provide their services, if appropriate, in your office space. Along the same lines, you can provide healthy cooking classes in your office for your patients and charge them a small fee to attend. Try to come up with ways to make things like this as easy as possible for your patients...and don't be afraid to charge money for these services. Never underestimate what you think someone will pay if it makes their life easier and it ultimately helps them.

3. **Nutritional Supplements**. Many doctors in private practice have acknowledged the positive role that

dietary supplements play in their patients' lives. This being the case, they have decided to provide and sell supplements from within their practices. Now, this might not be your "cup of tea" but it's definitely something to consider if you've never thought of it before.

It will require some research on your part (you'll definitely want to find and provide supplements that you trust) but once you've decided on the supplements that you would like to carry, it's pretty easy to get signed up as a distributor for those products and make recommendations to the patients that need them.

Americans spend nearly $40 billion annually on alternative medicine. Let's face it, you can either provide these items for your patients to purchase in your office or they will simply go and buy them somewhere else.

Two things that sell...Beauty and Sex!

On the other side, we have cosmetic and elective procedures that continue to grow in popularity. With very little research and with minimal training (depending on the service), you could be set up in your office to provide these services in no time. Once your training (if required) is complete, your patients can experience:

1. Laser and light opportunities
2. Neuro-toxin opportunities
3. Filler opportunities
4. Chemical exfoliation and peels
5. Fat reduction opportunities
6. Non-invasive body sculpting
7. Sclerotherapy
8. Hyperhidrosis
9. Other innovative elective procedures

[Please keep in mind that all of these, including the diabetes management, weight-loss counseling, and supplement sales, can be incorporated into the direct care model as well.]

Chapter 11

GETTING REFERRALS

This is perhaps an area that you typically don't think about but it's one of the key elements of a thriving practice. It's important, whether you maintain your traditional private practice or decide to convert to a direct care model, because a steady flow of referrals can be the lifeline that you need.

No need to worry...

Now, if you're considering converting to a direct care model and your current patient panel is anywhere from 2,500 patients up to 4,000 (or more) patients, you shouldn't have to worry about getting referrals. This is because you can expect to convert approximately 300 patients (on the low end) of your current patients to your direct care model. With these numbers, and depending on your revenue targets, you may or may not need additional patient referrals.

I'm sure you're familiar with the concept and accustomed to getting referrals from doctors...but the patient referrals I'm referring to here are not referrals from your colleagues but referrals from your current patients. *[Do you think I used the word "referrals" enough in that last sentence? =)]* Your current patients can and will provide additional, high-quality patients to your practice if you need them...but you'll have to ask.

Ask and you shall receive

You see, just like in any business, the best recommendation comes from someone who is already using the services. If you're new to an area, you would ask someone for a recommendation for a good dry cleaners, for example, as opposed to going out and trying different dry cleaners for yourself. If your dry cleaners had an active referral program, and you had a new friend who had just moved to town, you'd be inclined to tell your friend about your dry cleaners.

The same holds true for doctors' private practices...although you very rarely see a doctor with an active patient referral program. An "active patient referral program" means that you and/or your staff let your current patients know that you are actively looking for new patients. An "active patient referral program" also means that you incentivize the referral - so you would offer a Starbucks gift card or movie tickets or free services or anything you can imagine – to your patients who referred other new patients to your practice.

Be careful who you ask though

The thing to remember here though is that you only want to ask for referrals from your current patients that you enjoy treating. As the old saying goes, "birds of a feather flock together." And the patients that you enjoy treating - the patients that show up for their appointments and are on time, the patients that follow your directions, the patients that take their medications, etc. - these patients, more than likely, have friends like them and they are a great source of potential new patients for you.

Conversely, asking for referrals from patients that you do not enjoy treating will only get you...well...more patients that you don't enjoy treating. So be prudent!

Asking your patients a simple question, such as "Do you know some people who could benefit from the kind of care I offer?" and a low-cost brochure letting your current patients know about your referral program would do the trick nicely.

No pressure whatsoever

We're not talking about a "hard sale" here or coming across as desperate... nothing like that. What we're trying to do is make sure your current patients are aware of your referral program and make sure they're aware of the process they need to go through should they wish to refer someone (and the little "goody" they'll get when they *do* make a referral). The problem, in most cases, is that current patients don't know that you're looking for more patients and they certainly don't know the process for referring new patients to your practice.

Give this referral program a little thought, start an active patient referral program, make sure your current patients know the process, and you'll be pleasantly surprised by the new patient referrals they bring in for you.

Take advantage of the trend

For doctor-to-doctor referrals, as the direct care trend continues to rise, there will be more direct care doctors looking to refer their patients to other direct care doctors (as necessary). Some direct care doctors may need to refer their patients to a specialist and for obvious reasons both the patient and the doctor want that specialist to be a direct care specialist.

Alternatively, one of your direct care colleagues has a patient that is moving across town – to your neighborhood – and it would be inconvenient for them to continue seeing their current doctor. In this situation, because you're a direct care doctor closer to the patient's new location, it would be more appropriate for you to start following the patient. You would get this referral.

Be sure to get involved

There could also be a scenario in which a doctor in traditional practice is converting to a direct care model and during the conversion process he has more patients than he can comfortably accommodate. In this situation the doctor would be looking to make a referral for his excess patients to another doctor practicing the direct care model. The "doctor-to-doctor" referral examples above point to the importance of being involved in, and a member of, a group or association specifically for doctors following a direct care model. The **American Academy of Private Physicians**

105

(www.AAPP.org) is one such organization which has a strong network and useful resources, including annual conferences, which you're sure to find helpful.

Chapter 12

TUTORIALS

How to Set Up a Google Adwords™ Account and Launch an Advertising Campaign

First, go to www.google.com/adwords and click on that big blue "Get Started Now" button that you see on your screen. The good news is that it won't get much more difficult than this as we continue. Next, click whichever radio button is appropriate, depending on whether or not you already have any type of Google™ account. Once you have either signed in or set up an account, you will need to set your time zone and currency. That part is self-explanatory.

Next, you're going to want to go ahead and click on the little blue link you see that says "Sign into your AdWords Account." After you've done that, go ahead and click on "Create your first campaign."

Things can get as complicated as you want them to here, but for now, let's keep it simple. Type a name for your campaign in the box you see. Something like "Looking for a Doctor?" (or whatever you think is best) should do fine. Now, there are a lot of settings here to choose from, but there are really only two you need to be interested in changing at this point.

Type your daily budget for this campaign into the box near the bottom, and then click the check boxes for "Extend my ads with location information" and "Extend my ads with a phone number." Enter the appropriate corresponding information, then click "Save and Continue."

The next step is to create the text for your ad and type it into the box that has been provided for that purpose. You will also need to type in the address of your office's website in that same section. Once you have done both of those things, Google™ will populate some keyword suggestions a little further down the screen. Click "add" to the ones you feel are most appropriate to the types of services your office offers, then click "continue to billing information." Here, you will set up the payment information that Google™ can charge for your ads.

Once you have set up the payment information for your campaign, the next step is to wait for Google™ to approve your ad. Once they have done so, you will get an email notifying you that your campaign is now up and running. You will then be able to log into your account to monitor its results.

How to Set Up a Microsoft AdCenter™ Account and Launch an Advertising Campaign

First, go to https://adcenter.microsoft.com and click on "sign up." Fill out the sign up form, then click "submit." This next part is a little confusing. When you click "submit," the system is going to take you back to the home screen. At this point, you might think you did something wrong and your registration didn't go through...but it did. You just need to use the login details you just provided to sign in to the account you just created.

Now that you have set up your Microsoft AdCenter™ account, the next step is to create (and launch) your first advertising campaign. To get started, click "create campaign." After you fill in your budget, you're going to want to narrow down your ad targeting to people looking for doctors' offices where you're actually located.

To do that, click on "locations." Next, click on the radio button next to the words "Selected cities, etc." Type the name of your state into the search box that will then be provided. Press enter, then click "include" next to your location.

Type in your web address and the text of your ad in the next section. After that, you'll need to set up your keywords. In order to keep this process as simple as possible, you should let Bing™ itself make some recommendations for you here.

To do that, click on "research." Bing™ will then analyze your website and populate a list of keywords it thinks are relevant. Click to place a check mark in the box next to every keyword you want to target and then click the "add" button. Bing™ will then automatically populate per-click bid recommendations, which are set to be as low as possible, while still getting your ad displayed on the first page of results.

If you agree with the logic, and more importantly the *amount* Bing™ has used to calculate these bid recommendations, you need to accept them by clicking the "save" button at the bottom of the screen. Leave everything on the next page the way it is, then click "save and add billing."

After providing your payment information, there will be a short waiting period while Bing™ approves your ad. You will be notified when it starts running.

How to Set Up and Maintain a Facebook™ Business Page

The first step is to log into your Facebook™ account. You can even use a personal Facebook™ account as a starting point. If you don't already have a Facebook™ account, then you will need to create one by visiting www.facebook.com, clicking "sign up," and following their self-explanatory process. Once you've logged into your account, look for the word "Pages" on the left side of your screen, and click "more." Next, click the button that says "Create a page." Since your business is a doctor's office, the best category to click is "local business or place." Health is the category, so choose that and then fill in the rest of your details.

Now that you've filled in your information, click to indicate that you agree to the Facebook™ pages terms and conditions, then click "Get started." Upload a picture you want to represent your office. This could be a picture of the building itself or even a photo of the entire staff. Click "save photo" then enter an informative description of your office and its web address. Click the "yes" radio button then click "save info." It will suggest a Facebook™ web address for you. If you don't like it, you can change it. Then, click "Set address." For now, skip enabling the ads.

Next, Facebook™ will run you through a quick tutorial about how to finish getting your page up and running. Since that's what we're doing now, you can just keep clicking "skip" until you get through all of that. There is a lot you can change about your page as time goes on, but for now you will at least want to add your office hours and perhaps expand the description of the services you provide. Click "edit page," then click "update info." That will get you to a form where you can easily do both of those things.

You should have everyone in the office with a Facebook™ account "like" the page to get the ball rolling in that regard. While they are at it, they should invite all of their friends and family members to "like" the page as well. They will know what all of that means. By way of maintenance, it is just a matter of posting interesting content from time to time. Various health tips and news tidbits would be great. You might let your patients know about your page, too, so they can "like" it as well. If anyone else posts content on your page, make sure to interact with them.

How to Launch a Facebook™ Advertising Campaign

Once you have set up a Facebook™ page for your office, the next step will be to launch a Facebook™ advertising campaign. Log into your account and click on "ads manager." Next, click on "Create an ad" - it's the green button in the upper right hand corner of your screen. A great thing to advertise with your first Facebook™ ad is your Facebook™ page, so select it from the list you see. Next, click "see advanced options." Don't worry, we're still going to keep it simple, but we need to click that option in order to have the opportunity to advertise on a pay-per-click basis.

By advertising on a pay-per-click basis, you'll only be charged when your ad is clicked instead of being charged every time it is displayed. That way, you know you are getting something for your money. This is similar to the way Google™ AdWords charges for its ads.

Once you have entered the text and chosen the image you want to use for your ad, we're ready to proceed. Under "stories about your page," uncheck all of those options. They do not serve our purposes here. The next two boxes are the most important ones, so we are going to spend some time on them.

Most likely, your patients will live in the same county as your office, but you may want to leave this targeting as wide as your state (but probably not). Basically, you have the option of geo-targeting your ads – meaning, you get to choose the geographic area of the people you want to see your ad. You will want to advertise to people who are eighteen or older (typically) and you will want to include both genders. Since you are advertising a doctor's office, that's probably as narrow as you're going to want to get with your advertising. By setting those parameters, you are making sure that you are not wasting money on clicks from youngsters or people who live too far away from your office to become patients.

Next, name your campaign and set up its budget. Now, you're going to do something extremely important. Select "optimize for clicks," then select "manually bid for clicks." You can actually bid a per-click price lower than Facebook's™ suggestions and I recommend you do that. Whatever Facebook's™ lowest recommendation is, I recommend that you bid half of that. This strategy has always gotten me great results and saved me a lot of money. I believe it will do the same for you.

Click "Place Order" and your ad will be submitted to Facebook™ for review. You will be able to log back in to your account to check and see if your ad has been approved.

How to Set up a Twitter™ Account and Make a Tweet

When you are at www.twitter.com setting up your account, it will ask you for your full name. You should use the doctor's name and the main business email of the office. Enter a password, then click "create my account." It will ask you to set up a user name. I suggest you keep this short and simple - reflective of the name of the doctor's office. Check or uncheck the two boxes based on your preferences, then click the big yellow button at the bottom. Unless you have some other people in the medical world you want to follow, you can just click "skip" at the bottom of the screen until you get to the point where you can upload a picture.

Once you have uploaded a picture, you will be ready to compose your first tweet. However, before you do that, you should go ahead and log into the email account you used to sign up for Twitter™. In your inbox, you will see an email from Twitter™. Go ahead and open it. In that email, there will be a button to click in order to confirm your email address. Go ahead and click on it. You need to do this so that you will have access to some of the Twitter™ features which you will be using later on.

When you compose your first tweet (which you can do by typing into the box in the upper left hand corner of your screen when you log into Twitter™) you will need to be concise. After all, you're limited to 140 characters. You will also need to be relevant. Health tips and interesting health news items are going to go over well, as will announcements of any changes at your office. Remember, you can also include links in your tweets where the people who read them can get more information. The link will automatically be shortened to twenty characters for you.

Eventually, someone will tweet you directly. As long as it is a relevant tweet, you should tweet them back. If they provide information you think your other followers will find interesting, it is nice to re-tweet them too. Your patients will really like that. They also like it if you follow them. So make sure you "follow back" any real people that follow you, especially if they are your patients.

The point of Twitter™ is to communicate with your patients. You can let them know things about your daily activities and things that are going on in your practice. The more your patients feel like they know you, the stronger your relationship will be with them.

How to Set Up a LinkedIn™ Account and Launch an Advertising Campaign

LinkedIn™ is similar to Facebook™, except that it is geared more toward professional networking than to simple socializing, as is the case with Facebook™. Since professionals are very likely to enter into a direct financial relationship with you, it is a very good place for you, as a direct care doctor, to establish a presence. To get started, visit www.linkedin.com. Fill in the form, then click the yellow button that says "Join Now." Fill in the next form as well and then click "Create my profile." On the "grow your network" screen, click "skip this step." You can come back and grow your network later.

Your next step is to confirm your email address, so go to your email inbox and do that. Then, when you get back to LinkedIn™, if you have already set up Facebook™ and Twitter™ accounts for your office, you should share with your friends and followers the fact that you are now on LinkedIn™ by clicking the appropriate buttons. You will probably grow your network on LinkedIn™ just by doing that. Next, choose whether you want a basic or premium plan. You might want to go with basic first in order to familiarize yourself with the platform and decide whether or not to upgrade later on.

During the next several steps, LinkedIn™ will ask you a series of questions in an attempt to help you flesh out your profile. Just keep typing the answers to the questions into the boxes provided or click "skip" as appropriate. You will also have the opportunity to upload a photo during this part of the process and you should certainly do that. Once you get to the yellow "done" button, you'll be ready to launch your first advertising campaign. As you will see, like so many things, advertising on LinkedIn™ is very similar to advertising on Facebook™.

In the upper right hand corner of your screen, you will see the words, "ads by LinkedIn™ members." Click on those words. Click on the big yellow button that says, "Start now." On the first page, you can enter the text for your ad, the web address, and a picture. Having done that, click "next step." Here, you can choose your targeting options, then click "next step" again. (Everyone on LinkedIn™ is already at least 18, so you probably just need to target to your specific state.) Leave all the other settings alone and just enter your budget on the next page. I suggest the minimum bid. Click "next step" one last time, then enter your payment info.

You are now ready to advertise on LinkedIn™.

How to Set Up a PayPal™ Account and Use it For a Recurring Billing Service

The first thing you'll need to do is go to www.paypal.com. After you've done that, you'll want to go ahead and click the blue "Sign up" button in the upper right hand corner of your screen. The next step is to click the yellow "Get started" button underneath "PayPal™ for business and non profits." Here you will be given the opportunity to choose your service option. I recommend the standard plan – so the next thing you should do is click the blue "Get started" button beneath that option.

At this point, PayPal™ wants to make sure that you understand you've chosen an option intended for use by people who don't already have an account. Since you already understand that, go ahead and click on "Create new account." You'll actually have to click on it twice to get to the form you really need. Once you've done that, the form is self explanatory. Fill it out and click on the orange "Continue" button at the bottom of the screen. From here, the sign-up process is very similar to that of any other website, including the standard email confirmation.

Once you have completed the steps outlined above, sign into your account. You will now be ready to set up your ability to use PayPal™ for recurring billing payments for your office. Click on the "Merchant Services" tab and click on "Create payment buttons for your website." Click on the big blue "Create a button" button and then choose "Automatic billing" from the drop down box. Click on the orange "Learn more" button and you will be taken to a page where you can sign up for this additional service.

It will cost you a monthly fee of $19.99, but it's well worth it as there a number of things you can use it for. Signing up for it after you have clicked on the red "Sign up now" button is even easier than signing up for PayPal™ in the first place...which you've already done.

The goal here is not to send your patients to the website to sign up for your recurring billing service but rather to give you and your staff a place to go and input the credit card details for your patients who are converting to your new direct care practice. You can, however, send your patients to fill in their own credit card details (if you like) once your webmaster has installed the PayPal™ button on your website.

Additionally, once you compare PayPal's™ fees to your current merchant service provider's fees, you may decide that you'd like to accept credit card payments in your office through PayPal™ - which you can do through the free electronic card readers they provide.

Chapter 13

ABOUT THE AUTHOR

Scott Cartwright, MPH

Scott R. Cartwright is the founder and Chief Executive of Health Priority, LLC – a healthcare consulting and marketing company in San Diego, CA. Scott helps you, as a doctor, with the "business" and marketing side of your practice so you can make more money, see less patients, and practice medicine on your terms.

Scott, a prior Naval Officer and Naval Aviator, has over 17 years of experience as a marketing (both online and offline), public relations, and sales expert. He also has over 11 years of experience in the healthcare field. He has worked directly with patients, with doctors in medical practices, and in a major hospital within a large health system.

Scott's marketing efforts have been seen and featured on websites such as Mayo Clinic, Walmart Labs™, WebMD™, About.com, iHealth™, and MedHelp™ to name a few. Additionally, he can help you create passive, recurring revenue from the knowledge you have acquired through your many years of medical training.

Scott holds a Bachelor's degree from Emory University in Atlanta, GA and a Master's degree in Public Health from San Diego State University in San Diego, CA. His concentration for his graduate degree was in Health Management and Policy. Scott is a San Diego native and he, along with his beautiful wife and son, continues to live in San Diego.

If you feel like you and your practice could use a little help, give Scott a call. He loves working with practices to help them make more money and provide better care to their patients! Of course there's no charge to talk to Scott or for him coming up with some ideas that will help you.

Promise: *You won't get any sales pitch or pressure from him of any kind...ever!*

Scott can be reached at 858.255.1612 or at his personal email address: scartwright@ehealthpriority.com.

www.ingramcontent.com/pod-product-compliance
Lightning Source LLC
Chambersburg PA
CBHW062023200326
41519CB00017B/4898